HOW I LOST 45 POUNDS IN 3
MONTHS JUST
BY CUTTING OUT SUGAR

How to lose weight
By

sugar Detox Diet

Dr. Sarah Colin

Seasonal Recipes & Exceptional
Ideas

BEST SELLER AUTHOR

Contents

- Faux Potato Salad
- Shrimp, Zucchini, and Wilted Kale Noodle Salad
- Mexican Cole Slaw
- Entrees
- No-Sugar Italian Marinara Sauce
- Eggplant and Goat Cheese Lasagna
- Tomato, Garlic, and Mozzarella Chicken Breasts
- Italian Deviled Chicken with Tomato and Eggplant
- Chicken Thighs Roasted with Lemon and Fennel
- Ground Turkey with Quinoa, Kale, Tomatoes, and Mushrooms
- Slow and Easy Pork Chops
- Spicy Pork Pot Roast
- Easy Fisherman's Stew
- Easy grilled salmon
- Mustard Braised Short Ribs
- Slow Cooker Short Ribs with Ancho Chili
- Mexican-style mini meatloaves
- Vegan-friendly Lettuce cups with Roasted Onion and Guacamole
- Vegetables and Side Dishes
- Roasted Cauliflower
- Cauliflower Mashed "Potatoes"
- Coconut Lime Cauliflower Rice

Introduction

When was it that sugar became our enemy? Oh, sure, back in the good old days our parents might have warned us not to eat too much candy, or all our teeth would fall out. And in our teens, we were told that too much soda would make our face break out and we would get fat. But then we would get a lollipop if we were good at the doctor's office, and our dentist would reward us for a good checkup with a certificate for a free ice cream soda. Talk about mixed signals!

Nowadays, though, dentists reward their stellar patients with a free toothbrush and a pack of sugar-free gum, and pediatricians will hand out superhero stickers. But there are still some old-school docs who continue to offer the good old lollipop as a reward (or consolation) to a child after a checkup and a shot. Well, it's only one lollipop, after all, and it does help little Johnny feel better. Again, mixed signals. No wonder so many adults have sugar issues.

Over the past few decades, since about the 1970s, people in the U. S., as well as most of the Western Hemisphere, have been showing signs that there is too much sugar in their diets. In fact, the average man/woman on the street usually takes in about 126 grams of sugar on a daily basis. When you consider that the American Heart Association recommends a maximum of 37.5 grams, or nine teaspoons a day, for men, and 25 grams, or six teaspoons, for women, it's plain to see that many of us are going way overboard with our sugar intake.

Our love affair with sugar has led to some very undesirable side-effects. The truth is, recent statistics show that 69% of Americans are overweight. That's more than two out of three! You can see the results of this growing (pun intended) problem everywhere you look. People are finding it more and more difficult to button a shirt, zip up a pair of pants, or bend over to pick up something they dropped. And, let's face it, it can be very painful when you have to buy a size (or two) larger.

With the continuing concern about our national pastime of eating too much sugar, the sugar police have sprung up everywhere, alerting us to the evils of refined sugars and processed foods, and flashing their warnings about the health problems associated with these evil food villains. These warnings carry a crystal-clear message: sugar can have all sorts of negative effects on our bodies. Here is just a partial list of some of the many health issues that sugar contributes to:

- Weight gain (that's a no-brainer)
- Diabetes (ditto)
- Heart disease
- Digestive problems
- Inflammation
- Chemical and mineral imbalances in the body
- Fatty liver
- Metabolic syndrome

- Nourishment for cancer cells
- Higher levels of "bad" cholesterol (LDL)
- Sugar cravings, even addiction
- Lower energy level and fatigue
- Brain fog
- Risk of developing or worsening depression
- Sagging skin and a greater tendency toward wrinkles (aka aging)

That's a long list, and it could be even longer. But it certainly does make a point: by cutting down our consumption of added refined sugars in our diet, we can crush our sugar demons and live a healthier, happier life. To help people reach the goal of controlling the amount of sugar they consume, a sugar detox diet is the best way to cleanse your body of the popular but problematic ingredient.

On an intellectual level, most of us understand that we'd be so much better off without sugar in our lives, but "detox" is such a scary word. It implies having to deal with cravings, withdrawal symptoms, deprivation, and other nightmarish associations. But remember, a sugar detox diet is temporary. You basically "reprogram" your sugar consumption so that you can continue on a path to a healthier lifestyle.

By utterly eliminating sugar, as much as possible, for a specific length of time, our bodies gradually reduce the craving for sugar.
Some programs suggest as very little as twenty-one, ten, even three days without sugar.

This book, however, can concentrate on a thirty-day ward, based on the premise that it takes more than three, ten, or twenty-one days to completely recalibrate your system
and your taste buds.
After these thirty days, you may now not be a slave to sugar, and you'll additional completely embrace a lifespan while not cravings and sugar-related health issues.

Of course, it's not going to be easy. Indeed, it is very likely that at certain points there will be withdrawal symptoms: headaches - especially if you're also having to give up sodas with caffeine, cravings, achiness, crankiness, perhaps even shakiness. But once all that toxicity is cleaned out of your system, you will clearly see that it has all been worth it.

So, what's so terrible about sugar, anyway?

Sometimes adults have trouble understanding where this problem with sugar came from all of a sudden. After all, sugar has been a part of our lives since childhood. We remember the birthday parties with plenty of cake and ice cream, the sweet rewards for a good report card, and the parental admonishments to "eat your vegetables, or you won't get any dessert. Tonight, its chocolate pudding." Ah, how much better we felt when the chocolate pudding made the disgusting taste of broccoli disappear.

But while children process sugar and get instant energy to keep them bouncing off the walls—and their parents' nerves—adults no longer have the capacity to utilize sugar in the same way as they did in their childhood years. All those decades of continuous over-exposure to sugar has broken down their sugar-processing capability so they no longer have what it takes to eliminate the overload of sugar. Even one seemingly innocent brownie might have them slumping drowsily over their desks thirty minutes after they eat it, fighting to stay awake.

For most of us, our nervous system tends to break down as we age, and our endocrine system tilts out of balance. That's the system of glands that controls the hormones that regulate body functions. Our growth, development, and metabolism rely on the hormones to be in perfect working order. When sugar interferes with these hormones, your body can find itself facing some unsafe, even dangerous, challenges.

What happens when you eat too much sugar

It's important to keep in mind that you're not aiming for zero sugar in your diet forever. Our bodies actually must have a certain amount of complex sugars to give us energy and fuel for our brain. But on the side of evil, sugar causes a release of dopamine in the brain, the same chemical that makes cocaine addictive. Our brain recognizes sugar as a reward, we get a temporary feeling of euphoria, and we want more. And more. And more. That's when the problems start. So, while sugar is a necessary element of our diet, it should remember its proper place.

Some experts suspect that sugar can be as addictive as cocaine or morphine, and studies on rats have actually resulted in withdrawal symptoms. Human studies, however, have at this point not provided sufficient data to show that there's a connection between sugar and addiction, but there is plenty of anecdotal evidence to show that addiction is actually possible. Just ask anyone who has experienced sugar withdrawal.

How the body processes sugar

When we consume an acceptable amount of sugar, it's digested quickly, and converted to glucose, which our body uses for energy. Many people will often experience that famous sugar "high" or "rush." Any sugar that is not used for energy right away is stored as fat in cells specifically designed for that purpose. They're even called "fat cells." The more sugar we eat, the more fat has to be stored, and the bigger the fat cells have to become to accommodate it.

To illustrate, let's imagine a scenario where you over-indulge at a church social or office pot luck. For some of us, that's not a huge stretch of the imagination. As always, more people brought desserts than anything else, and they all look absolutely delectable! You can't be so rude as to only eat the healthy stuff and turn up your nose at the desserts that Carol and Abbie slaved so hard on (even a trip to Costco for a cheesecake is a form of slavery), so you have just a little bit of this and a little slice of that. Now your body has to deal with all that sugar.

Without diving into too much scientific jargon, what happens now is your pancreas is called upon to release insulin to act as a kind of escort to move glucose out of your bloodstream and into your cells. This controls the level of sugar in your bloodstream so that you don't become hypoglycemic (blood sugar is too low) or hyperglycemic (blood sugar is too high).

When a normal person's eating is under control, insulin's job is to take the glucose molecules that the body doesn't convert to energy and store them as glycogen in the liver and muscles. If there is more glucose in the system than it can handle, the molecules become triglycerides and are stored in the fat cells. Although most of us have a finite number of fat cells in our bodies, the fat cells themselves are very elastic and can expand. As more and more fat is stored in them, the fat cells become larger, and so does our body.

When everything is performing normally, a surplus of sugar leads to an excess of insulin. In other words, insulin has to be released into the bloodstream proportionately to the sugar so that the blood sugar level doesn't go too high. When there is too much insulin at work taking the glucose out of the bloodstream, the blood sugar level eventually falls too low, which causes that familiar crash and burn. Then our bodies tell us that we need more sugar, and we're usually more than happy to submit to its demands.

When elevated insulin levels become chronic, there is a higher risk of getting heart disease, some cancers, acne, and other health problems. There is even evidence that there is a link between high insulin levels and near-sightedness.

If we get to the point where we're continuously over-indulging on sugar, the pancreas becomes exhausted, and it can't produce enough insulin to deal with the overload. With no insulin escort, all that extra sugar stays in your bloodstream, feeling lonely and unneeded.

At that point, the sugar molecules look around for someplace to go and attach themselves to protein molecules, which carry them through your whole system so that they end up in every part of your body.

This combination of sugar and protein is the blueprint for inflammation. Now, inflammation is part of your immune system's strategy to defend against injury and disease, so by itself, it is not the enemy. When you suffer an injury such as a cut or sprain, or an invasion of germs that give you a sore throat, white blood cells race to the site of attack and rally together to overpower the bacteria. It's a battle at first, and there will generally be some heat, redness, and swelling around the area, but this is a sign that the immune system is working to heal tissue cells.

But when inflammation becomes chronic, it can be the source of many health problems, tissue damage, and premature aging. In the case of uncontrolled sugar consumption, the immune system senses danger when too much insulin or those glucose/protein cells start flowing through your system. This raises the alarm that unwanted cells are roaming around in the bloodstream. The white blood cell soldiers speed to protect you from those supposed invaders, et voila! You have general, chronic inflammation.

When the inflammation goes on and on because of continued sugar consumption, you can easily end up with permanently damaged tissue as well as premature aging. To take the problem a step further, inflammation can occur anywhere in the body, restricting the walls of your blood vessels. When it occurs in the area of your heart, you have an increased risk of heart attack and stroke.

And then there's that other sugar, fructose

Fructose is a sugar that occurs naturally in fruit, but it also links up molecularly with glucose in table sugar, which is also known as sucrose. That's a lot of "oases," but it's an excellent way to identify hidden sugars when you're checking food labels.

Glucose and fructose are metabolized by the body in completely different ways. The metabolic processing of fructose occurs only in the liver, rather than through the bloodstream, so there is no release of insulin. In addition, there is a decrease in the production of leptin, the hormone that alerts the brain to tell you that you've had enough to eat. So if you ever have the feeling that you're still hungry, in spite of just completing a heavy meal, it's because there's not enough leptin to send your brain the message that you're actually not starving.

Fructose also produces more fat in comparison to glucose and actually seems to act more like a fat than carbohydrate in the body. In fact, in the opinion of many experts, fructose is the main suspect in America's growing obesity problem, which some are calling an epidemic. Since high fructose corn syrup (HFCS) bounced onto the scene back at the beginning of the 1970s, it has become the preferred sweetener in almost all non-diet sodas, as well as in many other processed food items. It has to be more than just coincidence that the upsurge in obesity began at about the same time.

Because fructose does not trigger the release of insulin and leptin, it's more likely that you will overeat when you're consuming fructose-containing foods. And when you're drinking your favorite monster-sized soda pop from the neighborhood quickie store, we're talking about as much as 186 grams of sugar, or even more. In an article, she wrote for Reader's Digest ("9 Offensively Enormous Beverages"), Lauren Gelman puts it into laser-sharp perspective: KFC's 64 0z. Pepsi, with its 217 grams of sugar and 780 calories, is "the caloric equivalent of a KFC Honey BBQ sandwich, a house side salad with ranch dressing, macaroni, and cheese, Associate in Nursing [*fr1] a turnover." That's tons of calories, particularly after you think about that it's simply a portable.

Now, granted, most people aren't going to polish off an entire gallon of Pepsi in one sitting. It might take an entire day. Even so, it's most likely not going to be the only calorie consumption of the day; in fact, without the appetite inhibiting effects of insulin and leptin, you're probably going to want to eat even more calories throughout the day. Too many days like that, and it's bound to have an effect on your body.

Recently, clinical, scientific, and animal studies have led to the conclusion that fructose has more damaging health effects on the body than glucose. Since the majority of fructose metabolism occurs in the liver, it becomes problematic because when your liver has to deal with too much fructose, it leads to a tsunami of metabolic disorders, including obesity, prediabetes or type 2 diabetes, fatty liver disease, and inflammation over the whole system. Keep in mind that fructose is not the only culprit in causing these problems, but the correlation between the introduction of HFCS and the escalation in the cases of obesity and these other health problems just can't be ignored.

Brain function

Adding insult to injury, more recent studies have indicated that too much fructose over an extended period of time not only affects your body, weight, and organs, but in adolescents, there was also a significant effect on the brain. In tests on rats, the ability to learn and remember was substantially lower in the pre-adult rats who ate a diet high in fructose. The results seem to carry over to pre-adult humans who consume quantities of drinks sweetened with HFCS; testing has shown that their brains don't function with the same efficiency and they are less able to remember important information.

Now that you're sufficiently outraged at what fructose can do to your brain and your body, you're probably all set to swear off all fruits and vegetables, right?

But let's not be hasty here. Although fruit and vegetables are a source of fructose, you have to consider that it's in its natural state, not in the concentrated form of HFCS or fructose as an added sweetener. When you eat whole fruit, (once you have finished the detox program) you are also getting important fiber, vitamins, and minerals, as well as antioxidants. Antioxidants are important in curbing the free radicals that tend to try to take over when you're on a diet high in sugar.

Of course, that's not to say that eating an apple doesn't spike your blood sugar level to some degree, but it's minimal compared to the empty calories of table sugar and sweetened processed foods. Nevertheless, you may want to back off of fruit to get your detox going, and once you have broken your addiction, go back to eating fruit as part of a healthy diet.

Dangers of sugar addiction

According to an article at the website yogabody.com, "Sugar itself is not the problem—we all need sugar. The problem is we're uptake it perpetually, morning till evening.
The poison is in the dose." Note the use of the word "poison." That pretty much puts the dangers of too much sugar in a pretty scary spotlight. Everyone knows that poison kills. But many of us fail to recognize that too much sugar can also be deadly.

We've already mentioned the negative effects sugar can have on your insulin levels, but let's dig a little deeper into what that actually means. Most people are aware of the association of high levels of insulin and diabetes, but there is also a dangerous connection to cardiac problems. If your insulin levels are continuously elevated, studies show that you have an increased risk of developing heart disease.

In fact, according to Julie Corliss, executive editor of "Harvard Heart Letter," one 15-year study concluded that people who ate a diet where their daily calories from sugar amounted to 25% of their total calories were over two times more inclined to die from heart disease compared to people who had less than 10% added sugar in their diets.

The other major danger factor connected to sugar addiction is inflammation. Although refined sugar, with its empty calories, is a poor food choice for humans, bacteria thrive on the energy that sugar provides. As the sugar feeds the harmful bacteria in your stomach, your immune system responds with its go-to survival strategy, inflammation. Now there is the potential of having to cope with even more discomforts and diseases such as indigestion and Irritable Bowel Syndrome.

Even more sobering, a recent study indicates that there may even be a connection between elevated insulin levels and the development of Alzheimer's disease. And, as we mentioned earlier, there is evidence that sustained high insulin levels are connected to some types of cancers, which as we know, often lead to death.

But other diseases can also potentially become a problem as well because when you eat too much sugar, your immune system is significantly impaired so that you lose about 50% of your ability to fight against any invading bacteria or viruses. You are not only more likely to get ill, but you'll also have trouble getting over an illness quickly.

Could you be addicted to sugar?

Whether or not there's conclusive scientific evidence that sugar addiction exists in humans, there are definitely tell-tale signs that are dead giveaways that you have a problem with sugar. If you experience five or more of the symptoms on this list, you most probably have a dysfunctional relationship with sugar.

- Frequent cravings
- Feeling hunger even after you've had plenty to eat
- Turning to sugar as consolation when you feel blue or troubled
- Eating sweets when you don't even feel hungry
- Feeling embarrassed or ashamed about the way you eat
- Feeling fatigued or experiencing brain fog after eating
- Finding it difficult or impossible to lose weight
- Not being easily satisfied when you eat sweets
- Eating sweets until you're full to the point of discomfort
- Going back for more sweets, or even bingeing
- Hiding evidence such as candy wrappers
- Finding it difficult or impossible to cut back on sweets
- Eating as a substitute for a social life or activity
- Feeling a need for a sweet dessert after a meal

Why Detox

Now, granted, a full-out detox is pretty extreme, and you may be wondering why you can't just gradually back off of sugar. Well, if you've never tried it before, it might work. But for most of us, even a little bit of sugar is going to set off the cravings monster. If you continue to have the mindset that you need to satisfy that craving, it's going to be a very long time before you can pronounce yourself free of your sugar demons.

Detox is hard, no question about it, but it puts you in the proper frame of mind to say ABSOLUTELY, POSITIVELY NO! when your brain starts begging you to give in and just have one chocolate chip cookie or half of a Snickers bar. When you totally commit to cutting out all added sugar for thirty days, you're automatically setting yourself up for long-lasting success.

Why? Because it's the fastest, most effective way to take the sugar out of your system and completely retune and recharge your body chemistry. A detox will also reset your taste buds so that overly sweet foods just won't be as appealing. You will be able to start out fresh with a whole new arsenal of healthy eating habits that will lower inflammation and elevate your degree of general wellness.

Most importantly, you can say bye-bye to your addiction to sugar and refined carbs. According to Dr. Mark Hyman, author of the book Blood Sugar Solution, it's possible to see results after a 10-day sugar detox. In a recent study of 600 participants, after 10 days they observed that they were not troubled as much by fatigue, stress and anxiety, pain in their joints, digestive problems like acid reflux and irritable bowel syndrome, migraine headaches, and even skin rashes.

So, if 10 days without sugar will do all that, why go any longer? It's because we're human, and humans tend to backslide in the short term. After 10 days, reintroducing sugar to the system doesn't always go smoothly. The brain's affection for that sweetness is still pretty fresh, and it's too easy to revert back to the food we remember as making us so happy not that long ago. That's why the greatest success is achieved by persevering for the entire 30 days.

What a sugar detox can do for you

If you've read this far, you already have a clear idea of how a sugar detox will change your life for the better. A sugar detox will take your body back to its natural balanced state where your blood sugar levels, insulin levels, hormones, and metabolism are right where they should be. But just to reinforce your determination, here is another list; this time, it's an inventory of all the ways your well-being will revive once you are not always looking for the next sugar fix:

- You'll experience a dramatic increase in energy
- Your sleep patterns will improve
- Your blood pressure will go down
- You'll digest your food more efficiently
- You'll notice that your mood is generally better
- You'll lose weight and your body will have more lean mass
- Diabetics will have a reduced need for insulin
- Any joint or back pain you may have will disappear or be significantly diminished
- Your skin will look better, and younger
- No more brain fog
- You'll lower your risk for depression and anxiety
- You'll be better at sports and athletic activities
- Your thyroid will work more efficiently
- You're likely to experience illness less frequently
- Your heart will be healthier
- You'll experience fewer if any cravings for unhealthy food
- You'll enjoy an improved sex life

You may even get richer because you'll be saving money on doctor visits and expensive feel-better remedies!

Of course, all of these good effects aren't going to happen right out of the gate. The first few days of detox are likely to make you feel pretty miserable as the toxins leave your body and you experience withdrawal. There's even a name for this feeling: it's called a "healing crisis." Some people describe experiencing symptoms similar to having the flu. You'll probably want to give it up but hang in there. These symptoms will only last a few days, and the benefits you'll enjoy the rest of your life will be well worth a few days' discomforts.

How you should eat during a detox

The foundation of this specific sugar hospital ward diet consists of quality proteins, non-starchy vegetables, and healthy fats.

Below are lists of foods and beverages that you should include, limit, or avoid on your sugar detox diet:

The good guys:

Proteins

As you detox, in fact, most of the time, it's recommended that you start out your day with a generous helping of protein. Protein is your ally in keeping sugar cravings under control because it's slower to digest, so it helps you to feel full a bit longer. Quality proteins include all non-processed meat, eggs, fish, and shellfish. While dairy products are also a good source of protein, they do contain lactose, which is sugar. While you're detoxing, it's better to avoid dairy.

Non-starchy vegetables

Vegetables are an excellent source of fiber, which creates that full feeling and helps you to feel satisfied. Fiber reduces the absorption of fructose in the digestive system, helping to avoid spikes in your insulin levels. Make plenty of fresh salads out of seasonal leafy greens and dress with a spritz of fresh lemon juice, vinegar, and oil, or a delicious sugar-free salad dressing (see recipe section).

Besides leafy green vegetables, be sure to include plenty of the other kinds of vegetables as well, as long as they're the non-starchy, non-sweet type (peas, corn, carrots, etc.). Substitute cauliflower for mashed potatoes or rice, and you won't even miss those high-starch bad guys.

Instead of feeling deprived on your detox, take the opportunity to be adventurous and explore vegetables you've never tried before, such as fennel (which has its own therapeutic properties), daikon radish, and other veggies you may have been afraid to try until now.

Healthy Fats

Yes, in case you haven't heard, there is such a thing as healthy fats. These are the unrefined fats that come from animals, such as meats, eggs, and dairy products, which we focused on under protein. But there are also some plant-based healthy fats such as avocados, olives, tree nuts, seeds, and some non-tropical oils. These fats are identified as saturated or mono-unsaturated fats and provide omega-3 fatty acids, which have become well-known contributors to all kinds of health benefits.

Be aware, however, that there are other oils on the unhealthy fats list. These include vegetable oils that many of us have been using, unaware that they are harming us. Oils such as corn, canola, peanut, soy, and safflower are heavily refined, and they are high in omega 6 fatty acids, which have a tendency to contribute to inflammation.

Healthy fats will help you in your detox program by helping to eliminate your cravings and keeping you from feeling empty. You can always reach for a handful of almonds when you feel yourself sinking. You can also use nuts as a butter, ground into flour, or as an extra source of protein in a smoothie. Walnuts are an especially good choice for their health benefits, but you can also include brazil nuts, macadamias, pistachios, almonds, pecans, and hazelnuts.

Seeds also have many health benefits. Recommended seeds include hemp, sunflower, flax, chia, pumpkin, and sesame. For a health boost any time, you can add seeds to salads, soups, casseroles, smoothies, and other dishes.

What can you drink?

If daily sodas or diet drinks have been a part of your addiction, you're probably feeling pessimistic about your beverage choices. Maybe you've never enjoyed drinking plain water because it was so flavorless and flat-tasting. But don't despair; it's possible to jazz up regular tap water, or better yet, purified water so that it's refreshing and satisfying.

Additions such as mint sprigs, cucumber slices, grated ginger, and lime or lemon slices are great for giving water a flavor punch. Once you've finished the detox program, try adding some frozen berries or a cube of frozen watermelon to add a bit of sweetness without getting too much actual sugar. If you still miss the sparkle of your soda, invest in one of those machines that carbonate your water for you. Pretty soon, you won't even miss those sugary sodas!

Along with water, you can also drink unsweetened coffee or tea, unsweetened almond milk and coconut milk, club soda, mineral water, and seltzer.

How about condiments?

Condiments can be tricky, but as long as you are familiar with the ingredients, you should be fine. Feel free to use any herbs and spices; if you want to try one of those spice blends, check the ingredients to make sure there is no trace of sugar lurking in the jar. Other safe condiments are mustard, homemade ketchup (there's one teaspoon of sugar in a tablespoon of store-bought ketchup) capers, some salsas, and hot sauce, fish sauce, tomato paste, mayonnaise, sugar-free salad dressings, vanilla, and apple cider, white, or red wine distilled vinegar.

The bad guys

This is the part that could be a bit painful, but remember, the pain is only temporary. These are the items that you will have to take out of your life as you focus on your sugar detox.

- All types of sweets
- All types of sodas, including diet
- All types of caloric or non-caloric sweeteners, including honey, agave, and syrup
- Fruit juice
- Beer, including lite
- Cocktails (some spirits are included on the limited list)
- Products made with white flour, including bread, cereals, crackers, pasta, pastries, etc.
- Starchy vegetables such as corn, white or sweet potatoes, yams, plantains
- Canned or dried fruit
- White rice
- Margarine and other butter-like spreads
- Processed foods, including jarred pasta sauces, barbecue sauces, soups, etc.
- Multi-ingredient protein powder

Somewhere in between

These are the foods that you can eat in very minimal portions a few times a week. For most of them, it's best if you can wait until you get past the first three days so that they won't sabotage your progress. Then, if you seem to have your cravings under control, you can use these foods as an occasional treat, if needed.

- Legumes (lentils, beans, chickpeas)
- Fresh fruit in season (berries, lemons, and limes don't need to be limited)
- Whole grains such as quinoa, buckwheat
- Wine
- Alcohol with no sweetened mixer (vodka, gin, whiskey, or tequila)
- Dark chocolate (no, it's not on the bad guy's list, but remember to enjoy it only occasionally and very moderately)

On your mark, get set . . . preparing for your detox

This new way of eating is going to mean a big change in your life, so before you get started, there are a few things you should do to prepare. Once you're organized and focused, it will be much easier to stay on track and make it to the finish line.

It's always a good idea to check with your doctor before you begin any detox or cleansing program. If you are a woman who is pregnant or nursing, you definitely should not attempt to detox. Diabetics or people who are taking certain medications may also have a problem with the restrictions on this plan, as well as extreme athletes.

Set a goal to follow the rules on a day-to-day basis: avoid eating the foods on the bad guy's list and be careful to limit yourself on the moderation list. Try to eat mostly organic foods so that you don't complicate the detox process by sending unnatural chemicals into your body. Make sure that you are getting a generous supply of nutritious high fiber foods as well as plenty of water so that you can help your system process all those toxins out of your body. Since you will be repairing the damaged cells in your body, consider taking a vitamin and mineral supplement to help move that process forward.

Clean out your pantry and refrigerator. Read labels and toss out or give away (don't eat) anything that lists any type of sugar in the ingredients label. (Note that sugars may be listed under the nutrition facts, even though there is apparently no sugar in the ingredients. This is because sugar occurs naturally in many foods. Unless it shows a high number of grams of sugar per serving, it doesn't count as added sugar.)

Plan ahead so that all your shopping and eating is centered around the success of your detox journey. The more meals you make yourself, the more control you have on keeping unwanted sugar out of your body. Make sure to have plenty of viable options for meals and snacking around the house. Don't be that person who has nothing available to eat and then starts feeling so crazy they take a ten-minute drive to one of those places that sell those unhealthy smoothies – the kind with ice cream.

Be careful with your timing. Don't start your detox two days before the big cocktail party, and certainly don't try to start it during the holidays.
If you are not already on a regular exercise program, this is a great time to start one (again, check with your doctor). You can start by simply walking briskly through your neighborhood, or you can join a gym or take classes. Water exercise is very gentle on the joints, and you can try more vigorous exercise such as Zumba or aerobics. Yoga is also good. But use caution; if you start to feel light-headed or dizzy while exercising, you're probably overdoing it.

Try meditation to keep you focused on your goals and gain power over food cravings.

Get some social support. If there is no one you know who would like to go on this detox journey with you, at least enlist some of your family members or friends to be your cheerleaders and spur you on if you feel yourself beginning to weaken.

Don't give up! If you slip off the plan for some reason, just acknowledge that you're human, after all, and keep going. (If you lapse for a period longer than three days, you may have to go back to the beginning.

But bear in mind, it'll all be worthwhile within the finish.)

Your 30-day detox meal plan

There are many different programs out there for detoxing from sugar addiction. A few, like the Paleo plan, are much more rigid than the one described in this book. For our purposes, the first three days are the strictest, and the most difficult, and then the program gradually becomes gentler and kinder as you move from one phase to the next. By the end of the thirty days, your body should be ready to thrive on a whole new way of eating.

The kickoff: days one-three

Hopefully, you've followed all the instructions for preparing for your detox, so you are ready to dive in now with your mind, body, and soul. These first three days are not for sissies. The best way to attack this detox is cold turkey, no added sugars, no dairy, no grains, no starchy or sweet vegetables, no fruits, and no alcohol. Stick to the basics: nondairy protein, non-starchy vegetables, and healthy fats.

Start each day off on the right foot by eating a high protein breakfast. You can enjoy two or three eggs, any way you like (try scrambled with some chopped peppers, mushrooms, and onions) or you can make one of the high protein smoothies you'll find in the recipe section of this book. For your beverages throughout the day, choose water or unsweetened black coffee or tea. Green tea is especially good for its antioxidant properties, and many herbal teas are also beneficial, as long as they have no sugar in them. Remember, no juice.

For lunch, a mixed green salad with six ounces of chicken or salmon should hit the spot. If you're a vegetarian or vegan, you can go the tofu route. At dinner time, you can eat a slightly larger portion of meat, poultry, or fish and have some steamed green vegetables or another salad to go with.

It's important that you don't allow yourself to feel hunger pangs during this time because once you start feeling like you're starving to death, nothing is going to satisfy you, and you are more likely to just give up this whole thing. So eat small snacks when you start to feel a little hungry, and that should get you through the day.

For snacks during these three days, about an ounce of nuts can be very satisfying, or you can have celery and pepper sticks with some hummus. Since chick peas are on the list of items to limit, try making hummus out of cauliflower, beets, or other vegetables for a new flavor experience.

Once you've made it past the first three days, you'll probably start to notice interesting flavors that had previously been overwhelmed by the sugar in your diet that was getting most of your attention. Food that seemed bland before will pop with more flavor, and fruit will taste like dessert. This shows that your taste buds have begun to adjust and reset, and sugar is no longer king. Now you should give yourself a big pat on the back and move forward to day four.

Days four – seven

Beginning on day four, you can start to add some of the limited items to your food choices. Now you may have one apple as a snack or part of a meal (or dessert), as well as one dairy item such as half a cup of cottage cheese or plain yogurt or a slice of cheese. Don't go with the low-fat versions here, because fat, along with fiber and protein, is good because it slows down the way your body processes sugar. You can also indulge in a few high-fiber crackers, some of those higher sugar vegetables such as carrots and snow peas, and even a glass of red wine. (Limit yourself to three glasses of wine per week at this stage.)

Week two

Now that you've made it through your first week, the rest of the program should be smooth sailing. Any withdrawal symptoms you've experienced should be gone or going, unless you cheated and made some poor choices. Now, in the second week, you can add some berries and another serving of dairy. You can also say hello again to some of your old friends, starchy or sweet vegetables such as butternut or acorn squash and yams.

Week three

You're still plugging along! You have so much to be proud of, and you're probably really starting to notice a difference in your energy level and the way you feel! Now you can add more items to your program. Enjoy a bowl of oatmeal with cinnamon and berries for breakfast. You can also add some other grains, such as quinoa and barley. Include grapes and oranges in your fruit selection, and add one more glass of wine to your weekly allowance. As an extra reward, you may have up to one ounce of dark chocolate per day, but maybe by now you don't even feel you need it.

Week four

Are you starting to feel human again? Then week four will probably be heaven because now you can start putting a modest amount of starches back into your plan, including whole grain bread! This week you can actually have a slice of toast with your eggs or put make a sandwich out of your meat or fish. You can also make some rice to go with your stir-fry, and have an extra glass of wine per week for a total of five glasses. As you finish week four, you'll be in control of your sugar addiction and ready to maintain a lifestyle where sugar is an occasional, well-thought-out indulgence rather than a life-controlling, health-destroying tyrant.

Maintenance: how to live a low sugar life from now on

 As you complete your thirty-day program, you should be feeling like a brand-new person. This a good time to make a promise to yourself that you will never, ever backslide. That doesn't mean you can't treat yourself once in a while, as long as you do it mindfully. When there are ice cream and cake at a birthday party, go ahead and have a small slice of cake or a scoop of ice cream in honor of the birthday person. You're not addicted anymore, so you're the one in charge, not the sugar. Just remember that these indulgences should be occasional; if you get back into the pattern of eating sweets regularly, that old addiction, like Arnold Schwarzenegger in The Terminator, will "be back."

As you begin to reintroduce sugar into your life again, remember the daily limits recommended by the American Heart Association: no more than 25 grams for women, and 37.5 grams for men. That certainly doesn't leave you much wiggle room for added sugar. But you don't need to worry about the sugar that occurs naturally in fruits, vegetables, and milk. These foods have enough vitamins, minerals, fiber, and protein to make it possible for the benefits overcome the risk.

When you do feel the need to add some sweetening to a meal, avoid refined table sugar and use natural substitutes instead. Raw honey, molasses, pure maple syrup, pureed banana, dates or date sugar, and coconut palm sugar are all natural sweeteners that include important nutrients rather than just providing empty calories.

Another natural option is stevia. This is made from the leaf of a plant native to South America and is 200 to 350 times sweeter than sugar. Although it doesn't provide nutrients of its own, stevia does offer the benefit of adding sweetness without giving you more calories or raising blood your glucose levels, so you might like to try it out when you feel you need a little extra sweetness.

You can also explore turbinado sugar and sucanat– these sugars are actually made from the same sugar cane as table sugar, but they go through much less processing and no chemicals. As a result, they hold on to the nutrients of the sugar cane, which are lost in the processing of white sugar. Instead of sugary sweetness and empty calories, these sweeteners provide a more flavorful sweetness with a hint of molasses or caramel, as well as some vitamins and minerals that include iron, calcium, potassium, magnesium, manganese, phosphorus, niacin, and copper.

Both sucanat and turbinado are the natural tan color of the sugar cane because the molasses hasn't been processed out. Their granules are coarser than the granules of refined sugar, but they can be run through a food processor to make them finer and more suitable for baking.

Whatever natural sweetener you use, make sure to keep the daily limit in mind. If there is a question of how well your body will tolerate different sweeteners, try each sweetener by itself for two or three days to evaluate whether you have any problems with it. If you notice that you develop gas, diarrhea, or bloating, your body may have a problem with that food. Also be aware that changes in your energy level, your appetite, mood, or mental abilities could be caused by an intolerance to a food.

Once you complete a sugar detox, you can go back to eating any fresh fruits you like; you'll probably notice that fruit tastes fresher, sweeter, and more delicious than it did when you were a sugarholic. Continue to read labels for hidden added sugars, and avoid packaged, processed food and items containing white flour. Dark chocolate is still your friend because of its ability to stave off cravings and help with high blood pressure, and seeds and tree nuts are still a great option for snacking.

What about cravings?

Although your cravings should be mostly under control now, life does happen, after all. Whether it's stress, joy, excitement, boredom, the blues, or just those old hormones, things go on that can trigger a craving. After all the hard work you've done, now is not the time to surrender. Don't be distracted by cravings. Stand up and mount your defenses.

Be your own therapist. Is this really a craving? Or is your inner child remembering how good it felt to have some cookies and milk in the afternoon after school? This mental desire for a treat is not a bona fide craving, and you should be able to get control by employing the good old mind-over-matter strategy.

Maybe you're just thirsty. Have a glass of water and wait a few minutes to see if the feeling goes away. Even if that isn't the problem, a little extra hydration never hurt anyone.

Or maybe you're tired. Having low energy doesn't mean you need to have a sugar fix. If you can, do some meditation or take a short nap. Or re-energize by going for a walk around the neighborhood or the building and get your circulation going.

How about a change of scenery? Boredom often leads to uncontrollable snacking. Take in a movie or do some window shopping. Just avoid the food court and the snack bar.

Get busy. If you have nothing to do, you can't stop thinking about your craving. Throw yourself into some challenging tasks at work or around the house.

Spend some time creating something fabulous that's not edible. Call a friend and talk about the current world situation. That should get your mind busy on something else besides your desire to eat.

If all else fails, you may be truly hungry.
Don't worry, it happens to the best of us.
At this point, denying your hunger will only make it worse, so go ahead and fix yourself a snack. But make sure it's a healthy one.

Sample recipes

The recipes in this section use a mix of different ingredients designed to satisfy your changing needs as you pass through the different phases of the sugar detox diet. As you select recipes, be aware of the ingredients and the possible substitutions so that you can pass through each phase of your diet with no complications.

Beverages and smoothies

Beet Coconut Water Detox
Yield: 1 serving
Coconut water is creating a buzz among the health conscious. It's a popular choice for hydrating because it has a low calorie count, no fat, and no cholesterol. What it does have is a healthy dose of potassium and other minerals, as well as electrolytes. There is a bit of natural sugar, though, so it's best to save this one for when you're further along in your sugar detox process.

Ingredients
- 1 medium size raw beet, peeled and coarsely chopped
- 2 cups chilled unsweetened coconut water
- 1 lemon, juiced

Directions
Put all ingredients into a blender. Pulse until liquefied. Garnish with a lemon slice.

Spiced Green Tea Tonic
Yield: 1 serving

This tonic is sure to perk you up when you feel you need a little push to get you past a low-energy point. Turmeric is a great anti-inflammatory because of its antioxidants, and cinnamon can help regulate blood sugar levels. You might want to try out other therapeutic and restorative spices (see Appendix A) so that this tonic will be good for whatever ails you.

Ingredients
- 1 green teabag
- ¼ teaspoon turmeric
- ¼ teaspoon cinnamon
- 1 cup purified water, near boiling (green tea leaves are delicate and don't stand up well to boiling water)

Directions
1. Place teabag in mug and add turmeric and cinnamon.
2. Pour in hot water and allow to steep for approximately 2 minutes.
3. Remove the bag and stir thoroughly to dissolve the spices.

Whole Food Protein Shake
Yield: 1 serving

This healthy protein shake is courtesy of Dr. Mark Hyman, author of The Sugar Solution. The protein comes from all the nuts and seeds, and it's a very satisfying way to start the day.

Ingredients
- 2 Tablespoons hemp seeds
- 2 Tablespoons chia seeds, soaked overnight
- 2 Tablespoons pumpkin seeds
- 2 Tablespoons almond butter
- 4 walnuts
- 3 Brazil nuts
- 1 Tablespoon coconut butter
- 1 banana
- 1 cup wild blueberries
- 1 cup water
- 1 cup unsweetened almond milk

Directions
Place all ingredients in liquidizer and method till sleek.

CALL it a Smoothie
Yield: 1 serving

The name is the acronym of the main ingredients:
Cucumber, avocado, lemon juice and lime juice.
CALL it refreshing!

Ingredients
- 1 Tablespoon lemon juice
- 1 Tablespoon lime juice
- ¼ cup ice
- ¾ cup cucumber, peeled, cut into chunks
- 1 Tablespoon mashed avocado
- 2 pinches sea salt
- 2 pinches black pepper

Directions
Combine all ingredients and method till sleek and
creamy.

Coconut Pumpkin Spiced Smoothie
Yield: 2 servings

Ingredients
- 1 frozen banana
- ¼ cup pureed organic pumpkin
- 1 cup coconut milk
- 2 teaspoons pumpkin pie spice
- 1 cup ice cubes

Directions
Combine ingredients in blender and process until smooth and creamy.

Breakfast

Omelet with Spinach and Mushrooms
Yield: 2 servings

An omelet is a great way to start any day. It may take a little time, but overall, it's pretty simple to prepare. You can enjoy this one with any of your favorite allowed veggies.

Ingredients
- 4 eggs, lightly beaten
- sea salt and ground pepper to taste
- 2 Tablespoons extra virgin olive oil
- 1 cup spinach leaves, coarsely chopped
- 1 cup cremini mushrooms or mushrooms of your choice, sliced

Directions
1.   Whisk eggs milk, salt, and pepper in a medium bowl.
2.   Heat the olive oil in a medium non-stick skillet and sauté spinach and mushrooms until spinach is wilted and mushrooms are tender. Drain any excess liquid and set aside.
3.   Add half the egg mixture to the skillet. As it starts to become firm, add half the spinach and mushroom mixture. Fold. Repeat for the second half of the egg mixture.

Cheesy Baked Eggs with Spinach
Yield: 6 servings

Eggs and spinach again, and why not? The combination can't be beaten for giving you plenty of protein and nutrients. This time they're baked in individual ramekins so everyone can have their own little casserole. For the early days of your detox, you can leave out the cheese.

Ingredients
- 4 teaspoons olive oil
- 12 cups fresh spinach
- 2 teaspoons minced garlic
- 1 cup shredded low-fat mozzarella cheese
- 6 eggs

Directions
Preheat oven to 350° F.
1. Place half the oil in a large skillet. Add 1 teaspoon of garlic and half the spinach and sauté for 2-3 minutes, until spinach is wilted.
2. Add 1/2 cup of cheese and stir to combine.
3. Spray 6 ramekins with nonstick cooking spray.
4. Separate the spinach-cheese mixture into 3 ramekins.
5. Heat the other 2 teaspoons of oil in your skillet; add garlic and the rest of the spinach and cook as before.
6. Separate among 3 more ramekins.
7. Carefully crack one egg into each ramekin on top of the spinach mixture.
8. Bake for 15 minutes. The yolks should be slightly runny.
9. Season with salt and pepper.

Frittata with Sun-dried tomato and feta
Yield: 4 servings

This egg dish is similar to an omelet, but there is no folding.

Ingredients
- 2 teaspoons olive oil
- 1 clove garlic minced
- 1/2 cup diced onion
- 1/2 cup sun-dried tomatoes, drained and chopped
- 2 eggs
- 1/2 cup egg whites
- 1/4 cup unsweetened almond milk
- 1/2 cup crumbled light feta cheese light
- 2 chopped scallions

Directions
1.   Heat oil over medium heat in an oven-proof skillet. Add garlic and onion, and cook until onion is tender and has lost its crunch.
2.   Stir in sun-dried tomatoes, and heat for 2-3 minutes.
3.   Place eggs, egg whites, and milk in a small bowl and whisk together. Pour mixture into the skillet and sprinkle the feta cheese evenly over the top.
4.   Reduce heat to low. Continue cooking on stove top until set around the edges and center is slightly runny.
5.   Move skillet to oven and broil frittata for 3-5 minutes. The frittata is done when the center is firm. Cut into pie slices and, if desired, top with more feta and scallions.

Snacks and Appetizers

Homemade slow cooker ketchup
Yield: about 2 cups

When you make your own ketchup, you can leave out the sugar that is such a major ingredient in store-bought ketchup. Using a slow cooker brings out the full, rich flavor of this recipe.

Ingredients

- 1 small onion, diced
- 2 granny smith apples, peeled and finely diced
- 2 cloves garlic, minced
- ½ teaspoon sea salt
- 1/4 teaspoon allspice
- 1/4 teaspoon cinnamon
- 1/8 teaspoon cloves
- 1/4 teaspoon ginger
- 2 tablespoons apple cider vinegar
- 1/4 cup water
- 6 oz. tomato paste

Directions

1. Combine all ingredients in a slow cooker. Set the cooker to low and let cook for 4 hours. Allow the mixture to cool slightly.
2. Place into a food processor or blender and blend until smooth. Do not over-fill the container, as the warm ingredients will tend to expand and may splatter out.

3. Once blended and silky smooth, place the ketchup into glass containers and allow it to come to room temperature before storing in the refrigerator.

Homemade ketchup may separate after sitting, so shake or stir before using. Since homemade ketchup is preservative free, plan to use it within a few weeks to avoid spoilage or mold.

Roasted Beet Hummus

Yield: about 1 ½ cups

This substitute for chickpea hummus isn't complicated, but it does take some patience since it takes 2 days for the beets to be ready! Use as a dip for pepper strips and celery, or spread on whole wheat toast when you reach that stage of the detox. Add a couple of slices of avocado for a meal or snack that's healthy, tasty, and pretty.

Ingredients

- 1 ½ cups beets, peeled and chopped into ¼ inch dice
- 1 cup of water
- ½ cup distilled white vinegar
- A solution of 1 cup water and 1 cup white vinegar
- 1/4 cup rice wine vinegar
- 2 Tablespoons balsamic vinegar
- 1 small jalapeno, seeds included
- 1 red chili pepper
- 3 cloves garlic

Directions

1. Place chopped beet pieces into the water/vinegar solution for up to 48 hours.
2. After marinating, remove beets and add to 1 cup of boiling water. Let simmer for 15 minutes. If you prefer the taste of roasted beets, another option is to place beets in a pan and oven roast at 350° F for 35 minutes.

3. Once cooked beets have cooled, place in a food processor or blender, add rice vinegar, balsamic vinegar, a jalapeno, chili pepper, and garlic. Puree until smooth.
4. If consistency is too thick, add some of the water-vinegar solutions until it has a pleasing texture.

Enjoy as a spread or dip with veggies, crackers, or toast. Can also be served with fresh avocado slices or feta cheese.
This hummus may be stored up to a week in the refrigerator.

Cauliflower Hummus

Yield: about 4 cups

Cauliflower is a healthy substitute for many things: potatoes, rice, and, as in this hummus recipe, chickpeas! There are some powerful flavors in this one!

Ingredients

- 1 head cauliflower (separated into florets, about 8 cups)
- 3/4 cup tahini
- 1/4 cup extra-virgin olive oil
- 3 Tablespoons lemon juice
- 6 cloves garlic
- 4 teaspoons cumin
- 1 ½ teaspoons sea salt
- 1 teaspoon paprika
- 1/4 teaspoon cayenne (optional)

Directions

1. Steam cauliflower florets for 5-7 minutes, until tender, but not limp.
2. While the cauliflower is cooking, place tahini into a food processor and process until it is light and fluffy, about 2 minutes.
3. Mash the garlic cloves, remove the skin, and cook in a small amount of olive oil over medium-high heat just for about 15-20 seconds, to release an aroma. Remove from heat.
4. Add the garlic to the food processor and pulse with the tahini until smooth. Place the steamed

cauliflower florets into the food processor, a few at a time,   and process until it begins to look smooth. 5.   Add the rest of the ingredients, pulsing until well combined.

Keep at room temperature for an hour or two to integrate the flavors. Then it may be stored in the refrigerator. Before serving, remove from fridge to come to room temperature (at least half an hour before serving). Serve at room temperature with your favorite vegetables or crackers on the side.

Artichoke Hummus

Yield: 4 servings

Whoever it was that first realized that there were edible parts on this very strange-looking plant deserves to have a statue erected in their honor! Artichokes are a tasty meal or snack unto themselves, or as ingredients in so many dishes, such as this no-chick pea hummus.

Ingredients

- 1 can artichoke hearts (14 oz.), packed in water, drained
- 1 clove garlic, minced
- 2 Tablespoons extra-virgin olive oil
- 1 Tablespoon fresh lemon juice
- ¼ cup tahini
- ¼ teaspoon ground cumin
- Salt and pepper to taste
- Finely minced fresh herbs such as parsley, basil, or oregano

Directions

1. Add drained artichoke hearts and minced garlic to the bowl of a food processor, process until coarsely chopped.
2. Add olive oil, lemon juice, tahini, and ground cumin. Process again until mixture has a smooth texture. Season with salt and pepper to taste.

Before serving, drizzle with a little more extra virgin olive oil and sprinkle with minced fresh herbs. Serve with crudités, pita chips, or crackers.

Savory Stuffed Mushrooms
Yield: 24 mushrooms

These little stuffed mushrooms are delightful as a pass-around at a party or a small snack or meal at home. If you don't like the flavor of rosemary, you can experiment with other spices to get the flavor that you like.

Ingredients
- 24 small/medium mushrooms
- 1 Tablespoon olive oil
- ½ cup finely chopped carrots
- ¼ cup finely chopped celery
- ¼ cup finely chopped yellow onion
- 2 cloves minced garlic
- ½ pound ground beef
- 2 finely chopped teaspoons rosemary
- 1 teaspoon of sea salt
- 1 teaspoon black pepper

Directions
Preheat oven to 375° F. Line a baking sheet with aluminum foil.

1. Wipe the mushrooms with a damp kitchen towel or paper towel and remove the stems. Using a spoon, remove the gills from the underside of the mushroom cap. Set prepared mushrooms aside.
2. With stove set to medium, heat olive oil and add carrots, garlic, onions, and celery, and cook until just starting to get tender.

3. Add ground beef, and combine and cook with sautéed vegetables. Continue to cook on medium high until the meat is nicely browned. Add the rosemary and stir. Drain off any fat.
4. Stuff the mushroom caps with the ground beef mixture, carefully place them on the foil-lined baking sheet, and bake at 375° F for approximately 10 minutes.

Allow cooling slightly before serving.

Salads and Salad Dressings

Balsamic Hummus Salad Dressing
Yield: about 4 servings
Salads are a great part of any healthy eating plan, but when you pour on sugary or fatty salad dressings, you virtually cancel out the benefits. This salad dressing recipe and the ones that follow not only taste delicious but they keep your salad healthy.

Ingredients
- 5 Tablespoons hummus
- 4 Tablespoons balsamic vinegar
- 2 Tablespoons extra-virgin olive oil
- 1 teaspoon garlic powder
- sea salt and pepper to taste

Directions
In a little bowl, whisk all ingredients until combined. Serve over tossed greens and vegetables

Creamy Avocado Salad Dressing

Yield: about 4 servings

This dressing does have a bit of natural sugar from the fresh-squeezed orange juice, but it's perfectly fine to have after the first three days of the program.

Ingredients
- 1 ripe avocado, pitted, peeled and chopped
- ½ cup extra-virgin olive oil
- Lime juice from 1 lime
- 3 Tablespoons freshly squeezed orange juice
- ½ teaspoon minced chives
- 1 Tablespoon cilantro, finely chopped
- sea salt and pepper to taste

Directions
In a blender, puree all ingredients until smooth. Serve over tossed greens and vegetables.

Creamy Lemon Herb Salad Dressing
Yield: about 4 servings

This dressing is tart, healthy, and 100% sugar-free.

Ingredients
- 1/2 cup hemp hearts
- juice of 1 lemon
- 1 Tablespoon. chopped cilantro
- 1 small garlic clove, coarsely chopped
- 1 teaspoon minced chives
- 1 Tablespoon chopped dill
- sea salt and pepper to taste

Directions
In a blender, puree all ingredients until smooth. If needed, add water for a thinner consistency. Serve over tossed greens and vegetables

Dang Cold Asian Noodle Salad
Yield: 4 servings

The recipe for this Asian noodle salad is courtesy of Guy Fieri.

Ingredients
- 1 teaspoon sesame oil
- 2 tablespoons of rice wine vinegar
- 3 tablespoons soy sauce
- 1 teaspoon hot chili oil
- 1 tablespoon hoisin sauce
- 5 tablespoons extra-virgin olive oil
- 1 carrot, thinly sliced or julienned
- 2 celery stalks, thinly sliced or julienned
- 5 green onions, bottom 4 inches, thinly sliced
- 1/2 cup thinly sliced napa cabbage
- 1/2 red bell pepper, thinly sliced or julienned
- 1/2 cup julienned bok choy
- 1 cup bean sprouts, optional
- 3 tablespoons minced fresh cilantro leaves
- 3 tablespoons sesame seeds, toasted, for garnish
- 4 tablespoons unsalted peanuts, for garnish
- 1 package soba noodles

Directions
1.   Boil water in a medium stock pot, add salt and cook noodles.
When finished, place noodles in an ice water bath to cool.
Drain and set aside.
2.   In a medium bowl combine sesame oil, vinegar, soy sauce, hot chili oil, hoisin, and extra-virgin olive oil.

Mix totally and so mix ready vegetables and noodles.

3. Garnish with sesame seeds and peanuts, if
    desired.

Faux Potato Salad
Yield: about 4 servings

For the uninitiated, faux is the French word for fake. That means there's not a single potato in this salad. Maybe it doesn't taste like the real thing, but it's still very tasty, very healthy, and very sugar-free.

Ingredients
- 1 pound cauliflower
- 1/3 cup plain yogurt
- 1 Tablespoon olive oil
- 2 Tablespoon white vinegar
- 1 Tablespoon Dijon mustard
- 1 teaspoon garlic powder
- 1/4 teaspoon paprika
- 1/4 teaspoon celery salt
- 1/4 teaspoon sea salt
- 1/4 teaspoon pepper
- 2 eggs hard boiled, chopped
- 1/4 cup chopped red onion
- 1/4 cup chopped scallions

Directions
1. Steam the cauliflower until fork tender, about 10 minutes. Cool to room temperature for 20-30 minutes. If you prefer the taste of roasted cauliflower, go for it!
2. For the dressing, place the next 9 ingredients in a bowl and whisk until well combined. Stir the dressing into the cauliflower and add in onion, eggs, and scallions.
3. Chill for 30 minutes or until ready to serve.

Shrimp, Zucchini, and Wilted Kale Noodle Salad

Yield: 4 servings

Ingredients

- 2 Tablespoon extra-virgin olive oil
- 4 cloves garlic, minced
- 8 ounces deveined shrimp, tails removed
- 1 bunch organic kale, stems removed, chopped (about 6 cups)
- 1 teaspoon salt
- 1/2 teaspoon pepper
- 1-pint cherry tomatoes
- 2 cups zucchini noodles
- Juice of 2 lemons (about 1/2 cup)
- 1/4 cup fresh basil, chopped

Directions

1. Heat oil in a large skillet over medium-low heat. Add garlic and cook just until soft.
2. Add shrimp and cook until curled around edges and both sides are pink.
3. Reduce heat to low and add kale, tomatoes, salt, and pepper. Continue to cook until kale is wilted.
4. Stir in lemon juice and zucchini noodles and cook for 2-3 more minutes until zucchini is firm/tender.
5. Serve topped with fresh basil.

Mexican Cole Slaw
Yield: 8 servings

Ingredients
- Bottom of Form
- 8 cups thinly sliced green cabbage
- 4 cups thinly sliced red cabbage
- (You can use all green or all red cabbage if you prefer)
- 4 green onions, thinly sliced
- 1 cup chopped cilantro (or more)
- 8 Tablespoons plain yogurt
- 6 Tablespoons fresh lime juice (more or less to taste)
- hot sauce to taste (about 1 teaspoon Tabasco sauce is good)
- salt to taste

Directions
1. Combine cabbage, green onions and cilantro in a large salad bowl.
2. In a small bowl, whisk together, yogurt, lime juice, and hot sauce.
(You might want to begin with but the complete quantity of juice and sauce and keep adding till you've got the required mix.)

3. Use a wooden spoon to fold dressing into cabbage mixture.
Season to style with salt and serve as a shot, or chill for a couple of hours.

Entrees

No-Sugar Italian Marinara Sauce
Yield: 8 cups or 16 servings

Store-bought marinara sauce and spaghetti sauce are big offenders when it comes to unexpected sugar. But then, many homemade sauce recipes also have a little of the white stuff in them to cut down on the acid of the tomatoes. This sugar-free recipe includes grated carrots to add a little sweetness and cut down on acidity.

Ingredients
- ¼ cup extra virgin olive oil
- 3 cloves of garlic, minced
- 1 onion, finely chopped (about 1 cup)
- 1 carrot, peeled and grated
- 2 (28 oz.) cans of crushed tomatoes
- 11/2 cup water (for richer flavor try half water and half red wine)
- 2 Tablespoons fresh oregano, minced (or one teaspoon dried)
- 1 ½ teaspoon dried fennel seed
- 2 Tablespoons chopped fresh parsley
- 1 teaspoon salt
- pepper to taste
- 1 teaspoon red chili pepper flakes
- fresh chopped basil and grated Parmesan cheese for topping (optional)

Directions
1. Heat the oil in a large pot or Dutch oven.

2. Sauté the garlic, onion, and carrot until onion is translucent.
3. Add all the other ingredients and bring to a boil.
4. Reduce heat to low, cover, and simmer for 25-30 minutes.

This basic recipe can be easily modified by adding ground beef or turkey, meatballs, mushrooms, or anything that strikes your fancy. Pour it over cooked spaghetti squash (or whole grain pasta once you've finished the detox), or use it for eggplant and goat cheese lasagna or chicken parmesan.

Eggplant and Goat Cheese Lasagna
Yield: 6 servings

This pasta free dish is a delicious way to use your homemade marinara sauce.

Ingredients
- cooking spray
- 1 large eggplant, sliced into ¼ inch discs
- 1 recipe homemade marinara sauce or spaghetti sauce
- 4 11 oz. log of goat cheese, sliced

Directions
Preheat oven to 375°. Spray cooking spray into a 9x13 baking dish.

1. Lay ¼ of the eggplant slices in a single layer in the bottom of the dish.
2. Cover with a layer of marinara sauce, and dot with ¼ of the sliced cheese.
3. Continue layering three more times with goat cheese layer on top.
4. Bake for 45 – 60 minutes, or until cheese is melted and sauce is bubbling.

Let sit for about 10 minutes before cutting into squares.

Tomato, Garlic, and Mozzarella Chicken Breasts
Yield: 4 servings

Ingredients
- 2 large garlic cloves, mashed and minced
- 2 tablespoons anchovy paste
- 1/2 cup finely chopped flat-leaf parsley
- 4 tablespoons olive oil, divided
- 4 boneless, skinless, chicken breast halves
- 2 large plum tomatoes, cut into slices
- 8 ounces of Mozzarella di Buffalo or Whole Milk Mozzarella cut into slices.

Directions
1. Stir together garlic, anchovy paste, parsley, 1 tablespoon oil, and 1/2 teaspoon freshly ground black pepper.
2. With a sharp knife, slice through the center of the chicken breasts horizontally, but don't cut all the way through. Spread them open like a fan, lay them flat on your work surface, and pat dry with a clean kitchen towel.
3. Spread parsley mixture over the surface of the chicken and fold chicken pieces in half, forming a pouch.
4. Insert the tomato slices and cheese into the pouch and brush the outside with oil, salt, and pepper.
5. Season the outside of the chicken breasts with 1/4 teaspoon salt and 1/4 teaspoon pepper, then brush with 1/2 tablespoon oil. If you'd like, use skewers to hold the chicken halves together.

6. Heat remaining tablespoon oil in a large nonstick skillet over medium-high heat until hot. Add chicken and cook about 2-3 minutes per side, or until nicely browned.
7. Lower heat and cover skillet. Continue cooking until chicken is done, about 5 more minutes. Reserve pan juices and serve on the side of the chicken.

Italian Deviled Chicken with Tomato and Eggplant

Yield: 4 servings

Ingredients

- 1 pound chicken thighs, skinless and boneless
- 3 Tablespoons extra-virgin olive oil
- Fine salt and black pepper to taste
- 1/4 tsp hot red pepper flakes to taste
- 2 small globe eggplants (could also use zucchinis), chopped in 1-inch chunks
- 1 yellow onion, sliced
- 2 garlic cloves, sliced
- 2 large tomatoes, cubed or 1 cup canned plum tomatoes, chopped with juice
- 3/4 cup chicken broth (be sure to check the label)
- 12 pitted Kalamata olives, halved
- 1Tablespoon capers, rinsed and drained.
- 2 Tablespoons corn starch mixed with 2 Tablespoons water
- 2 Tablespoons chopped parsley

Directions

1. Cut chicken thighs (or chicken breasts) into bite-sized pieces that will cook evenly. Heat 2 Tablespoons of olive oil in skillet and brown chicken on both sides. Transfer to plate and season with salt, pepper, and red pepper flakes.
2. Add another 1 Tablespoon of olive oil to the same pan and brown eggplant, onion, and garlic for 5 minutes until soft.

3. Return chicken to skillet, add tomatoes and stir. Add chicken broth, bring to a boil and simmer partially covered for 15 minutes.
4. Turn the chicken pieces over and add olives and capers, and cook for an additional 10 minutes or until chicken is cooked through.
5. Stir in corn starch mixture and simmer, stirring, until sauce thickens.

Chicken Thighs Roasted with Lemon and Fennel

Yield: 4 servings

Chicken thighs are so versatile you could probably have them a different way every day for a year! Try this recipe on your family, or even serve to company.

Ingredients

- 6 chicken thighs
- 2 small fennel bulbs
- 4 large garlic cloves, minced
- zest, and juice from 1 lemon
- 2 tablespoons olive oil
- 2 tablespoons dry white wine
- teaspoon kosher salt
- Freshly ground black pepper

Directions

1. Place oven rack in the center of the oven and preheat to 425°F.
2. Place the chicken thighs in a large bowl; set aside.
3. Cut the fronds and the ends of the stalks off the fennel bulbs, setting fronds aside. Slice each bulb into quarters and then slice into 1-inch-thick segments.
4. Chop about 1 tablespoon of the fennel fronds and add to the chicken along with fennel slices.
5. Add garlic, lemon zest, lemon juice, oil, and white wine. Season with salt and pepper and toss ingredients until well combined.
6. Arrange the mixture on a large cooking sheet covered with foil. The fennel should be placed

around the outside of the sheet and the chicken pieces should be close together in the center. Any juices remaining in the bowl can be poured over the chicken.

7.   Roast in preheated oven about 30 minutes, until the chicken is brown and crispy and no pink juices are running out. Internal temperature should be about 160°F. The fennel should be tender and slightly brown around the edges.

8.   Remove the pan from the oven and cover with another sheet of aluminum foil. Let sit for approximately 5 to 10 minutes, and serve.

Ground Turkey with Quinoa, Kale, Tomatoes, and Mushrooms
Yield: 4 servings

All these healthy ingredients cook up quick and easy, and all in one pan!

Ingredients
- 1 tablespoon olive oil
- 1 pound lean ground turkey
- one small yellow onion, thinly sliced, then halved
- salt and pepper to taste
- 1 pound mushrooms, sliced
- 4 cups baby kale leaves, tightly packed
- 2 cups chopped tomatoes (or use canned tomatoes)
- 3/4 cup dry white wine
- 3 cups cooked quinoa
- 1 Tablespoon fresh parsley, chopped
- 1 ½ teaspoon fresh oregano, chopped
- 1 ½ teaspoon fresh basil, chopped
- Parmesan cheese

Directions

1. In a large skillet, heat oil over medium heat. Add onions and cook until translucent. Add turkey, salt, and pepper.
Break up the turkey and cook till turkey is boiled through and brown.
Remove turkey mixture from pan and set aside.
2. Add mushrooms to pan, working in small batches if necessary. Sauté until golden brown. Add

tomatoes and kale to mushrooms and continue cooking until kale is wilted.

3. Increase heat to medium-high and add turkey and onion mixture. Add wine and bring to a boil. Lower heat and simmer until wine is reduced by about half.

4. Stir in quinoa and herbs and continue cooking until warmed through.

Serve with a sprinkle of freshly grated Parmesan cheese.

Slow and Easy Pork Chops
Yield: 4 servings

Slow cookers not only make our lives easier, but they also make meat juicier and more flavorful. If you've ever struggled to cook a tender pork chop, you have to try this recipe.

Ingredients
- ½ cup plus ¼ cup all-purpose flour
- ½ teaspoon ground mustard
- ½ teaspoon garlic pepper
- ¼ teaspoon seasoned salt
- 4 - 4 oz. boneless loin pork chops
- 2 Tablespoons olive oil
- 1 ½ cups homemade chicken broth

Directions
1. Place ½ cup flour, ground mustard, and seasonings in a large resealable plastic bag and shake until combined.
2. Add each pork chop to a bag, one at a time, and shake bag until pork chop is coated.
3. Heat oil in a large skillet over medium-high heat. Quickly brown pork chops on both sides. Move pork chops to a large (5 qt.) slow cooker.
4. Take remaining ¼ cup flour and whisk in chicken broth until smooth. Pour mixture into a slow cooker to cover pork chops. Cover, cook on low setting for 3-4 hours.
5. Remove meat to a serving dish and transfer cooking liquid to a mixing bowl. Whisk until you have a smooth sauce, serve on the side, or pour over pork chops.

Spicy Pork Pot Roast

Yield: 8 servings

Ingredients:

- 2 medium dried ancho chilis, stem and seeds removed
- 3 medium dried guajillo chilis, stem and seeds removed
- 2 bay leaves
- 2 Tablespoons cider vinegar
- 1 small yellow or white onion, coarsely chopped
- 3 cloves garlic, chopped
- 1 tsp thyme, marjoram or oregano (ideally a mix of all three)
- 1/4 tsp fresh ground allspice
- 1/4 tsp fresh ground cloves
- 1 1/2 Tablespoons vegetable oil
- 1/2 tsp Kosher salt
- 3 1/2 lbs. boneless pork shoulder or butt roast, or bone-in pork shoulder roast with some skin left on

Directions

1. Place the chilis in a small bowl, fill with hot water and let stand for 10-20 minutes to rehydrate. Put a heavy cup on top of the chilis to keep them submerged.
2. Transfer the chilis and 1 cup of liquid to a food processor or blender.
3. Grind the bay leaves, allspice and cloves with a spice grinder or mortar, then add to the blender along with the vinegar, onion, garlic, and mixed herbs. A process to a smooth puree.

4. If using a bone-in pork shoulder, make inch deep incisions all around the roast. If using a boneless cut, cut into slabs roughly 3 inches thick.
5. Place the roast in a large roasting pot and spoon or rub the chili paste all over, working into the incisions.
6. Pour the remaining cup of water around the meat, cover, bring to a boil, and simmer for about 2 1/2 hours.
7. Let the pork stand, covered, for about 20 minutes before serving. The meat should be fork tender. Remove the bone, shred, and serve.

Easy Fisherman's Stew
Yield: 4 servings

This stew, recipe courtesy of Elise Bauer of Simply Recipes, is pure comfort on a cold winter night, at a beach bonfire, or as a nice Lent-observant meal. You can also use your choice of shellfish if you like, but be aware that shellfish need a little more time to cook.

Ingredients
- 6 Tablespoons olive oil
- 3 large garlic cloves, minced
- 1 ½ cups chopped onion (about one medium onion)
- 2/3 cup fresh chopped parsley
- 1 ½ cups chopped tomato (or use a 14-ounce can of tomatoes, whole or crushed, with their juices)
- 2 teaspoons tomato paste (optional)
- 8 oz. of clam juice
- ½ cup dry white wine
- 1 ½ lb. firm white fish fillets, cut into 2-inch pieces
- (good choices are halibut, cod, red snapper, or sea bass)
- Pinch of dried oregano
- Pinch of dried thyme
- 1/8 teaspoon Tabasco sauce (or to taste)
- Salt and freshly ground black pepper to taste

Directions
1. In a large heavy pot over medium-high heat, heat olive oil, and add onion. Sauté for about

4 minutes, then add the minced garlic and cook an additional minute.

2. Add parsley, stir for 2 minutes. Stir in tomatoes and tomato paste, and allow to simmer gently for about 10 minutes.

3. Pour in dry white wine and clam juice, then add fish pieces. Return to simmering for about 3 to 5 minutes, until the fish is cooked through and flakes apart easily.

4. Add spices and Tabasco, and salt to taste. Serve in bowls.

Easy grilled salmon
Yield: 4 servings

Salmon has become well-known as a dish that's especially good for your health. The marinade in this recipe is simple to make, and it gives the salmon a delicious zing.

Ingredients
- •1 pound wild-caught salmon filet
- •1 teaspoon dried basil
- •1 teaspoon dried oregano
- •1 teaspoon black pepper
- •1 teaspoon salt
- •1/4 cup extra virgin olive oil
- •2 cloves minced garlic
- •Juice of 1 lemon

Directions
1. Rinse salmon under cold water, pat dry with a paper towel, and cut into 4 equal-sized portions.
2. Combine olive oil, fresh lemon juice, garlic, basil, oregano, salt, and pepper in a jar, place the lid on tightly and shake well to mix.
3. Place salmon in a baking dish, pour marinade overturning salmon to fully coat.
4. Place in the refrigerator to marinate 1 hour before grilling.
5. Preheat grill to medium-high.
6. Grill salmon 4 minutes on each side.

Salmon is medium once it flakes simply with a fork.

Mustard Braised Short Ribs
Yield: 4 – 6 servings

Another dish for a cold winter evening, or whenever. This rich, hearty meal will stick to your ribs without raising your blood sugar.

Ingredients
- 2 pounds boneless beef short ribs
- 1 tablespoon olive oil
- sea salt and pepper
- 4 cloves of garlic, mashed
- 3 cups natural beef broth
- 1 cup Dijon mustard
- 3/4 cup of your favorite unsweetened non-dairy milk
- 1/4 teaspoon sea salt
- 8-10 sprigs of fresh thyme

Directions
Preheat the oven to 325°F. Before braising, allow short ribs to come to room temperature.

1. Dry with paper towels and sprinkle all sides generously with sea salt and freshly ground black pepper.
2. Heat olive oil over medium-high heat in a large oven-proof Dutch oven.
3. Add the short ribs to the pan and cook for 3-5 minutes without turning, so that a dark crust forms on one side.
4. Repeat on all of the other sides of the short ribs.

5. The garlic cloves can be cooked alongside the short ribs until both sides are a golden brown.
6. Remove the short ribs and garlic to a plate.
7. Deglaze the pot by adding the beef broth and stirring with a wooden spoon, making sure to scrape up the bits at the bottom of the pan.
8. Whisk in the mustard, milk, sea salt, and fresh thyme until evenly combined. Allow the flavors to blend by bringing mixture to a simmer for 3 minutes.
9. Return the short ribs and garlic to the Dutch oven and cover with a lid. Place in preheated oven, for 2 1/2 hours.

Serve with a side of mashed or roasted cauliflower.

Slow Cooker Short Ribs with Ancho Chili
Yield: 4 servings

Succulent, savory with a little bit of a kick. Those are the words to describe this beef dish. Start your slow cooker in the morning so you'll have plenty of time to let this dish cook to its tender best. If desired, you may substitute a chuck roast for the short ribs.

Ingredients
- 2 Tablespoons olive oil
- Sea salt & coarse ground pepper
- 2 1/2 lbs. beef short ribs
- 1/2 onion, diced
- 2 cloves garlic, minced
- 1 Tablespoons ancho chili ground pepper
- 2 teaspoons oregano
- 2 teaspoons chopped chipotle peppers in adobo sauce
- 1 teaspoons salt
- 1 teaspoon pepper
- ¼ cup lime juice
- ¼ cup beef broth
- 2 Tablespoons tomato paste

Directions
1. Pat ribs dry and seasons generously with coarse salt and pepper.
2. In a skillet, heat olive oil at medium-high. Sear the ribs, one side at a time, turning with tongs as each side reaches a deep brown color.
3. For the last minute or so of browning, add the onions and garlic to the skillet to help caramelize the meat.

4. Transfer contents from skillet to slow cooker and add the rest of the ingredients.
5. Set slow cooker on low and cook about 8-10 hours, or until meat is completely cooked and fall-off-the-bone tender.
6. Remove ribs from slow cooker, shred the meat, and return to slow cooker to combine with the juices.

Serve as is, spoon over cauliflower rice or mashed cauliflower, or cool and add to salad.

Mexican-style mini meatloaves
Yield: 4 servings

You don't have to go south of the border to enjoy the distinctive flavors in these little meatloaves. But you can imagine yourself there as you feast on this fare, maybe with a cool glass of cucumber-mint water to go along with it.

Ingredients
For the sauce:
- ½ cup tomato paste
- ½ cup of water
- Tablespoons finely diced red bell pepper
- 2 teaspoons cilantro, chopped
- 1/4 teaspoon chili powder
- 2 pinches sea salt
- black pepper to taste
- For the loaves:
- 1 Tablespoon olive oil
- ½ cup finely chopped onion
- ½ Tablespoon grated garlic
- 2 eggs, beaten
- 2 pounds lean ground beef
- 1 teaspoon cumin
- 1 teaspoon coriander
- 1 teaspoon chili powder
- ½ teaspoon of sea salt
- ¼ teaspoon black pepper – or more to taste
- 2 carrots, grated
- 1 bell pepper, cut into very fine dice
- ¼ cup chopped cilantro

Directions

Preheat oven to 375°F.

1. Over medium-low heat, combine ingredients for the sauce in a small saucepan and simmer, stirring occasionally, for about 5-10 minutes. The consistency should be fairly dense, almost like ketchup. If the sauce reduces too much, add water 2 tablespoons at a time and whisk, until the desired texture is reached.

2. Meanwhile, using a medium skillet, heat the olive oil and sauté the onions over low to medium heat until they are translucent and slightly brown at the edges. Add the grated garlic, stirring for about a minute.

3. Place the ground beef into a large mixing bowl and add the beaten eggs, carrots, bell pepper, cilantro, and spices. Combine well.

4. Line 2 mini loaf pans with parchment paper and divides the meatloaf mixture between the 2 pans, pressing it in firmly. The meat will shrink a little bit during cooking, so it's fine if the mixture is slightly above the top of the pans.

5. Spread about 1/4 cup of the sauce evenly over the top of each loaf. The remaining sauce can be saved for dipping.

6. Bake uncovered loaves for 40-50 minutes, or to an internal temperature of 160°F.

Vegan-friendly Lettuce cups with Roasted Onion and Guacamole

Yield: 4 servings

Ingredients

- 2 large white onions cut into quarters
- 1 Tablespoon olive oil, extra-virgin
- 2 large, very ripe avocados, peeled, pitted and mashed
- ¼ cup of lime juice
- 1 red bell pepper, cut into fine dice
- 2 teaspoons finely chopped fresh parsley
- 2 teaspoons finely chopped fresh cilantro
- 1 clove minced garlic
- generous pinch ground cumin
- 1 large head Bibb lettuce, leaves separated
- 1 medium cucumber, diced
- 1 cup grape tomatoes, quartered
- 1 scallion, cut into very thin slices
- 3 Tablespoons chopped pecans
- 1 teaspoon sesame seeds
- Sea salt and freshly ground pepper to taste

Directions

Preheat the oven to 400°F.
Line an oversized baking sheet with a sheet of parchment paper.

1. Place the onions on the baking sheet and coat evenly with the oil, using your hands or a pastry brush.
1. Season with salt and pepper and roast for forty minutes.

2. To make the guacamole, combine avocado with the chopped pepper, cilantro, parsley, garlic, and cumin. Add sea salt and pepper to taste.
3. Working on a flat surface, add a portion of the roasted onions to each lettuce cup. Put a scoop of guacamole on top of the onions, and finish with tomatoes, cucumber, scallions, pecans, and sesame seeds.

Serve immediately.

Vegetables and Side Dishes

Roasted Cauliflower
Yield: 4 servings

Steamed cauliflower is great, but for a completely different taste, you have to try it roasted. It needs a little more attention, but you'll like the end result.

Ingredients
- 1 pound cauliflower (about one medium to large head), trimmed and cut into ¼ inch slices
- extra virgin olive oil
- sea salt to taste
- coarse black pepper

Directions
Preheat oven to 375°F
1. Place cauliflower in a large mixing bowl and drizzle with enough olive oil to coat all pieces. Season with salt and pepper, and toss.
2. Place cauliflower slices evenly on cookie sheet and drizzle with any remaining oil.
3. Bake about 25 – 30 minutes or until tender and caramelized on edges. Turn once midway through baking. Serve warm or let cool to room temperature. Delicious as is, or sprinkled with good aged vinegar.

Save any leftovers and add to a green salad

Cauliflower Mashed "Potatoes"
Yield: 4 – 6 servings

When you have a hankering for some mashed potatoes, but you know your body is better off without all that starch, cauliflower comes to the rescue again.

Ingredients
- florets from 1 head of cauliflower
- 3/4 cup water
- 2 tablespoons butter
- 2 tablespoons unsweetened non-dairy milk
- 2 teaspoons sea salt, + more to taste
- 1/8 teaspoon ground black pepper

Directions
1. Add the water and cauliflower to a large pot and bring to a boil.
2. Cover the pot and steam the florets over medium heat until they are easily pierced with a fork, about 15 minutes.
3. Drain and place cooked florets into a large food processor with the chopping blade inserted. Add the butter, milk, sea salt, and black pepper and process until the mixture looks like mashed potatoes.
4. Taste and, if necessary, add more seasoning, butter, or milk to suit your taste.

Coconut Lime Cauliflower Rice
Yield: 4 servings

This dish requires canned coconut milk, which you can get at most grocery stores. Avoid using the type that is packaged in cartons. It will need to be stirred well before you add it to the recipe.

Ingredients
- 1 head cauliflower, cut into florets
- 2 tablespoons extra virgin olive oil
- 1 yellow onion, diced
- 3 garlic cloves, minced
- 1 cup canned organic lite coconut milk, stirred
- zest and juice of 1 lime
- salt and fresh ground pepper to taste

Directions
1. Add florets to the bowl of your food processor and pulse until cauliflower looks like grains of rice. If you have a smaller-size food processor, work in small batches at a time so that the cauliflower doesn't turn into a paste.
2. Using a nonstick skillet over medium high heat, sauté onions in heated olive oil for 2 -3 minutes, until translucent. Stir in garlic and riced cauliflower; cook for 1 minute.
3. Add coconut milk and continue to cook for about 10 minutes, or until the liquid is absorbed.
4. Remove from heat; stir in lime zest and juice. Season with salt and pepper; style for seasonings and change consequently.

Garnish with chopped cilantro or parsley, if desired, and serve with lime wedges.

Charred green beans with crushed almonds
Yield: 4 servings

Just when you thought green beans could never be anything but boring, a new eating style helps you discover that you were so wrong. This recipe takes the waxy, blah green bean and turns it into a crispy explosion of flavor. The secret is in waiting until your oven is very hot before you char the beans.

Ingredients
- 1 pound green beans
- 1 ½ Tablespoons olive oil for cooking
- ¼ teaspoon salt, plus a pinch
- 1 ½ Tablespoons fresh dill, minced
- Juice from one lemon
- ¼ cup roasted almonds, chopped

Directions
Preheat oven to 400°F.
1. Drizzle olive oil over green beans and toss with salt.
2. Spread a single layer of beans on a large cookie sheet. (You may line it with foil for easier cleanup.) Be careful not to overcrowd beans.
3. When oven has reached the proper temperature, place the cookie sheet in oven and roast beans for 10 minutes.
4. Stir, flipping as many beans over as possible, then roast for 8 – 10 minutes more, until beans are blistered and charred.
5. Remove from oven and place in serving bowl. Stir in dill and lemon juice, and top with chopped almonds and a dash of sea salt.

Carrot Zucchini Fritters
Yield: 4 - 6 servings

When you're making vegetable fritters of any kind, a food processor is your best friend. Whip these fritters out in about a half hour, and enjoy your veggies! If you're in the later stages of the detox, you may even add a dollop of sour cream.

Ingredients
- 2 cups grated zucchini
- 2 cups grated carrots
- 2/3 cup almond flour
- 3 large eggs, lightly beaten
- ½ cup scallions, sliced
- Olive oil for cooking
- Sea salt and pepper to taste

Directions
1. Place grated vegetables in a bowl and sprinkle lightly with salt. Set aside and let the moisture come out for 10 minutes.
2. Using a clean dish towel or cheesecloth, press the vegetables to squeeze out as much liquid as possible.
3. Add eggs, scallions, almond flour, and seasonings to carrot/zucchini mixture. Stir until well mixed.
4. Heat olive oil in the pan over medium-high heat and spoon about 3 tablespoons of mixture per fritter into the pan. Press down with the flat side of a spatula to make a disk shape.
5. Cook in hot oil, turning once until both sides are golden brown.

Remove from pan and let drain on paper towels.

Serve with non-dairy sour cream, if desired.

Desserts

Sautéed Apples
Yield: 1serving

If you miss apple pie, this recipe for sautéed apples
will come to your rescue.

Ingredients
- 2 teaspoons butter
- 1 granny smith apple, peeled, cored, and
  sliced
- 1/4 teaspoon cinnamon
- 1/4 teaspoon mace or nutmeg
- pinch sea salt

Directions
1. In a small skillet, melt the butter over
   medium heat.
2. Arrange the apple slices evenly in the hot
   pan. Sprinkle with the cinnamon, mace and
   sea salt.
3. Gently stir to coat the apple slices with the
   butter and the spices.
4. Sauté for approximately 10 minutes, stirring
   occasionally, or until the apples have slightly
   softened.

Serve warm. Try it with a splash of coconut milk and
some extra cinnamon, if desired.

Chocolate Pudding with Chia Seeds
Yield: 4 servings

Yes, it's pudding. The sweetness comes from dates, so you're safe after the first 2 weeks.

Ingredients
- 2 cups unsweetened almond milk
- 1/2 cup chia seeds
- 1/4 cup natural creamy almond butter,
- 1/4 cup unsweetened cocoa powder
- 4 large dates, pitted and finely chopped
- 1 teaspoon pure vanilla extract

Directions
1. Place all ingredients into a bowl until thoroughly combined.
2. Move the bowl to refrigerator and chill pudding for 3 – 4 hours or overnight.
3. Transfer pudding to blender or food processor and process until creamy. If pudding is too thick, thin it with a little more almond milk.

If desired, top with chopped nuts or more chia seeds.

Tips on staying sugar-free

After completing the program, the main challenge will be for you to stay sugar-free as much as possible. Never take what you put into your mouth for granted, but be mindful of every bite. Thoughtless eating never did anything good for your health. When you realize that you are actually enjoying food that is not packed with sugar, it will make every meal a meaningful experience.

Continue to be vigilant as you shop for your meals, and keep the bad stuff out of your house and out of your life. Never stop checking those labels, and familiarize yourself with all the code names that sugar uses to disguise itself:

- Sucrose
- Glucose
- Lactose
- Dextrose
- Fructose (and, of course, high fructose corn syrup)
- Agave or agave nectar
- Brown rice syrup
- Evaporated cane juice
- Malt syrup

Remember to watch for these sugars on the ingredients list rather than the nutritional facts list. Of course, if the nutritional facts list indicates a total amount of sugar greater than the recommended number of daily grams, it's probably best to give that particular item a pass and opt for something else.

When the list of ingredients includes some of the natural sweeteners that we mentioned earlier, proceed with caution. Although they do have those nutrients that are unavailable in refined sugar, they are still processed in the same way by the body, so keep them to a minimum for the sake of your pancreas, liver, and all your cells.

Continue to be a planner. Do as much of your own meal preparation as you can manage so that you have no doubt about what you are putting into your body. Get your family on board your healthy lifestyle with you so that you don't have the burden of having to cook more than one meal at a time.

Get passionate about staying healthy, and implement some health-oriented rituals into your daily routine:

- Make it a morning habit to drink a beverage made from the juice of half a lemon stirred into a glass of warm or room temperature water. This will help eliminate toxins. It's even more effective if you use organic lemons and purified water.

- Drink plenty of water throughout the day, jazzed up with fruit and bubbles, if necessary.

- Have a daily smoothie full of fiber and nutrients, but no sugar.

- Keep the level of your blood sugar balanced by eating a small meal or snack every 2 to 3 hours. A few slices of apple with some sugar-free peanut butter or almond butter has both fiber and protein to keep you feeling satisfied.

- Be mindful of what you eat, how it tastes, and how it satisfies you.
- Try to include some raw food in your daily food plan. This shouldn't be too difficult since almost all fruits and many vegetables are best eaten raw. Cooking food isn't always the best choice health-wise since heat can destroy or diminish natural enzymes and nutrients.

- Nurture yourself. Spend quality time with friends and family. Enjoy a hobby or participate in a sport. Avoid stressful situations as much as you can, exercise, and meditate so that you will be healthy from the inside out.

You did it!

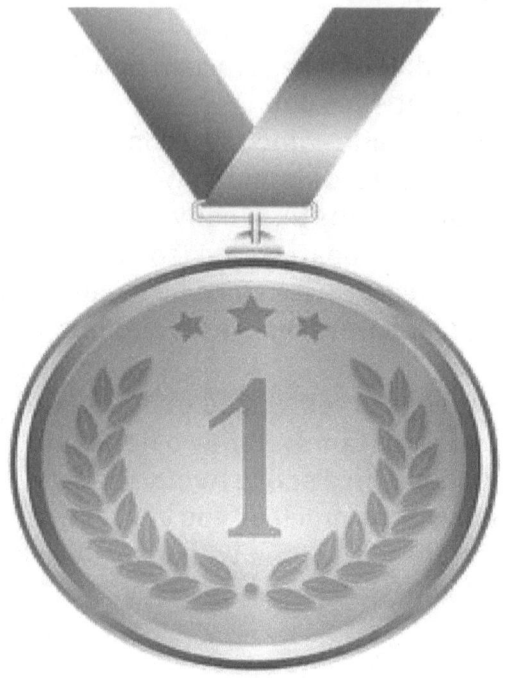

Congratulations! You have made it through this book, and hopefully through your own sugar detox program. You can justifiably declare yourself a winner in the battle against sugar addiction, and here is a virtual medal of accomplishment for you to virtually wear with well-deserved pride!

People who successfully complete a sugar detox program report that they feel much better than they ever imagined. Since they always depended on sugar to boost their energy, they're surprised at how energetic they feel without it. As your energy level improves, so will other aspects of your life: your sleep patterns, your skin, your moods, even your sex life. You won't experience those insane cravings anymore, and now it won't be a constant struggle to lose weight. While the process may have been a struggle, most people who go through a sugar detox program will tell you it changed their lives, and they suddenly find themselves looking forward to a much brighter future.

Here's to yours!

APPENDIX

Therapeutic and Restorative Herbs and Spices

This list of healthy herbs and spices should inspire you with ways to add them to your routine cooking or use them in smoothies and tonics to provide extra benefits that go beyond your low-sugar lifestyle.

Basil is an herb that has anti-inflammatory abilities, and it is also good for your cardiovascular system. Because it works to remove harmful bacteria from your system, it strengthens your immunity. It's used quite a bit in Italian cooking but is very good in all kinds of soups and other dishes. The flavor tends to be strong and sweet/savory/peppery.

Cardamom has antioxidants to fight free radicals and inflammation, and it is known to help with digestive symptoms such as heartburn and upset stomach. It has diuretic properties, which can help lower blood pressure. It has a delicious, spicy-sweet flavor that is commonly used in Indian cooking.

Cayenne pepper adds heat and spice to recipes, and, ironically acts as a calming agent to an irritated digestive system. Because of its cleansing properties, it is often part of many different detox plans. Its flavor is self-evident in its name: hot and spicy.

Cilantro is a natural cleansing agent to help purge your system of accumulated toxins from heavy metals. It also acts as a calming agent, and it can be used to improve sleep patterns. It has a fresh, tangy flavor that is commonly used in salsas and Mexican and Asian dishes.

Cinnamon is a very popular spice, so it's good to know that it also has some great health benefits. It can reduce cholesterol levels, and it also has anti-inflammatory and antiseptic properties, so it fights inflammation and infection. Cinnamon actually helps regulate blood sugar levels, so it's a great addition to a sugar detox diet. Additionally, it provides a metabolic kick to your system, so it can be an important addition to a weight loss program. Cinnamon tastes like nothing else, and it is great as a tea or added to the fruit.

Cumin is nutrient rich with important minerals such as potassium, thiamine, and, phosphorus. Besides giving you digestive benefits, it also helps lower the risk of getting diabetes. It's a savory, somewhat spicy flavor that most Mexican food-lovers are quite familiar with.

Fennel seeds are tiny little health machines. They provide a wide assortment of vitamins, minerals, antioxidants, and fiber. The health benefits include lowering LDL cholesterol (bad cholesterol) and defending against the risk of colon cancer. It can also help with weight loss and digestive problems such as acid reflux and flatulence. It has a licorice flavor and can be used as a tea or in cooking.
Ginger is well-known for its therapeutic benefits and is even being explored as a remedy in treating cancer. This is another spice with anti-inflammatory

benefits, so it helps to relieve various types of pain and digestive problems. Other benefits from this miracle spice include defense against bacterial and viral infections, improvement of cognitive functions, including memory and attention, and defense against Alzheimer's disease.

Ginger also helps to lower blood cholesterol and ease menstrual cramps. It has a very spicy flavor that is quite delicious when it's subdued by teaming it up with other ingredients.

Ginseng supports the immune system, and there is evidence that it also sharpens mental acuity and improves concentration. Ginseng is not generally used as an ingredient in cooking but is a popular daily supplement for many people.

Licorice root is known for its anti-anxiety properties and helping to control feelings of stress. It has a strong, unique flavor that people either love or hate.

Nutmeg is a good detoxifying agent, so it's frequently used in detox programs to step up the removal of toxins and impurities from the liver and kidneys. It has also been used to help with digestive upsets and sleep problems. It has a sweet, nutty flavor that's popularly used in baked treats and holiday egg nog.

Oregano, especially in its fresh form, is packed with antioxidants, fiber, vitamins, minerals, and some omega-3 fatty acids. Italian oregano is commonly used in sauces and other dishes, but there are several other varieties of oregano that cover a wide spectrum of flavors.

Parsley is more than just a decoration on your plate. It is a good source of antioxidants, and it contains vitamin C, to boost immunity and fight pain from inflammation, and vitamin K, which helps normal blood clotting. You also get B vitamins from parsley, which is good for your cardiovascular system and your heart health. It has a fresh, "green" taste, and it has a breath-freshening effect if you chew it.

Rosemary helps the immune and circulatory systems. Additionally, it has been shown to be helpful in soothing digestive troubles. It has a strong, somewhat minty flavor.

Saffron, in its extract form, has been shown to help with depression and PMS. It also seems to be a valuable aid in weight loss and appetite control. Note that these benefits are most associated with the extract, rather than the seasoning as it is used in cooking; therefore, care must be taken to avoid overuse, as side effects can occur. Pregnant women should not use saffron extract.

Sage is good because it contains antioxidants, and therefore has anti-inflammatory properties. It is often used in teas to soothe digestive complaints. The flavor is pleasantly bitter, but it can be overpowering when used in excess.

Thyme has potent antioxidant properties, which are beneficial by themselves, but there is also an anti-microbial benefit from consuming thyme. This quality helps keep harmful bacteria and fungi under control. It's a highly aromatic herb that has been described as having a lemony/peppery flavor.

Turmeric is great for its anti-inflammatory properties. Frequently used in Indian cooking, it has a distinctive, tart flavor.

Dear Reader,

Thank you for choosing to read my books out of the thousands that merit reading... I recognize that reading takes time and quietness, so I am grateful that you have designed your lives to allow for this enriching endeavor,
If you loved the book and have a minute to spare, I would really appreciate a short review on the page or site where you bought the book. Your help in spreading the word is greatly appreciated. Reviews from readers like you make a huge difference in helping new readers find subjects similar to

. I know you could have picked any number of books to read, but you picked this book and for that, I am extremely grateful.

I hope that it added value and quality to your everyday life. If so, it would be really nice if you could share this book with your friends and family by posting to Facebook and Twitter.

If you enjoyed this book and found some benefit in reading this, I'd like to hear from you and hope that you could take some time to post a review on Amazon. Your feedback and support will help this author to greatly improve his writing craft for future projects and make this book even better.

Thank you for your time!

Dr. Sarah Colin